The Biochemists' Songbook

The Biochemists' Songbook

By

Harold Baum

King's College
University of London

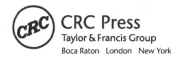 CRC Press
Taylor & Francis Group
Boca Raton London New York

CRC Press is an imprint of the
Taylor & Francis Group, an informa business

CRC Press
6000 Broken Sound Parkway, NW
Suite 300, Boca Raton, FL 33487

270 Madison Avenue
New York, NY 10016

2 Park Square, Milton Park
Abingdon, Oxon OX14 4RN, UK

Library of Congress Cataloging-in-Publication Data

Catalog record is available from the Library of Congress

Visit the CRC Web site at www.crcpress.com

To my wife Glenda
who still only nags me for my own good

PREFACE TO THE
FIRST EDITION

For some years it has been the custom that I write a biochemical song for our Departmental Christmas Party. The rules are that the song is written (to a well known tune) whilst travelling upstairs on the No. 22 bus between Putney Bridge and Manresa Road. Mrs. Stewart, our inspired Departmental Secretary, then transcribes the illegible scrawl into typescript, which is checked for biochemical rigour and for tolerable scansion by some of my long-suffering colleagues. The song is then duplicated and sung by everyone at the party, accompanied at the piano by another of my colleagues, Terence Steenson.

Some of these songs found their way to Sir Hans Krebs in Oxford, who very kindly encouraged me to continue producing them, and subsequently suggested (perhaps not too seriously) that I write an entire Introduction to Biochemistry in this format. My wife had been making a similar suggestion for some time, and the combined encouragement of two such remarkable patrons led to an increase in my scribbling activity —I began to compose on buses Nos. 85, 85A, 14 and 30 as well—and hence to the completion of the present collection. Consequently, only around half of these songs have so far been subject to the test of public performance.

However, on the basis of past experience I am confident that they all can be sung, provided that certain rules are followed. Firstly, the scansion must be worked over privately, as some words and phrases have to be accented at surprising places. Secondly, these are *songs*; they should *not* be declaimed as poems. Thirdly, they are intended for *communal* singing, preferably with musical accompaniment and ideally with a blood alcohol level of around 35 mg per cent.

Some of the songs may seem inordinately long—although no longer than some bar-room ballads I know. This is not really my fault; I didn't devise the pathways. In view of their length, however, I would strongly discourage any attempt to sing more than one a day.

If you have any difficulties in fitting the words to the music, or if you do not understand how the words relate to the pathways, please write to me and I will try to help. If you have suggestions to improve any of the songs, either for literary or biochemical reasons, please also write to me—just in case we produce a second edition.

PREFACE TO THE
SECOND EDITION

The first edition of my modest little songbook finally ran out of steam 13 years and several reprints after its first publication. I can only look back with astonishment at its popularity with students and professional biochemists alike. Indeed, in my anecdotage, I am now prone to tell true tales of having my songs sung back to me, in answer to questions at oral examinations, in places as far afield as the Medical School in Kuwait and the University of Nigeria, Nsukka. And it is also delightful to know that, among others, the Institute of Biophysics in the University of Moscow has used the book as a text in scientific English. Indeed, the only damage to my *amour propre* has not been lack of critical acclaim, but a tendency to be known internationally more for the songs than for my science.

Shortly after the book was first published, I began to receive polite letters pointing out, for example, that 'The Lincolnshire Poacher' is not a well known tune in Nagoya. So with the help of my brilliant musician friend Peter Shade, and masterminded by my awesomely energetic wife Glenda, we engaged the musical star Gary Bond to make a cassette of all my songs, except, for copyright reasons, the one on blood sugar. (There is another story, the gory details of which you shall be spared, of why the EMP song is less satisfactory than the others; briefly, the recording studio was struck by lightning during the final mix, by which time Gary Bond was on tour abroad.)

We offered the cassette for sale by mail-order, expecting to sell around 50 copies. Instead it became almost a cottage industry with nearly 2 000 copies being sold the first Christmas to purchasers in 60 different countries. Even now, so many years later, I still receive one or two orders a week, frequently on photocopies of ancient order forms.

But time moves on, and having now transferred the rights of the book to my good friends Taylor & Francis, (publishers since 1798, and whose early authors included Michael Faraday), a second edition is called for. For sentimental reasons, and also not to make the cassette redundant, I decided

ix

only to change one word in the original songs – 'glucagon' for 'adrenaline' in the (unrecorded) blood sugar song. This does not seem to be unreasonable. The pathways covered were so basic as to be essentially unchanged, notwithstanding that 13 years is such a long time in biochemistry.

Of course, if the songs were written anew there would have been G-proteins as well as glucagon, and the protein biosynthesis song would have been even longer. However, only the chemiosmotic song is now really wrong in detail, (although not in overall concept), and I'd like that one to stand as a clear statement of where Peter Mitchell's theory was in 1982. (Also that is one of the songs on the cassette where the accompaniment was a duet between Peter Slade and my dear late Uncle Micky, who was 80 at the time; and I'd hate to take that off the tape.)

Initially, I assumed that a second edition would require new songs, so I bought a new bus pass. But, sentimental fogey that I am, before I started to compose, I dusted off those Chelsea Biochemistry Department Christmas songs that were written after the first edition was assembled. Rapture! Not one of them was out of date, at least as far as they attempted to go in outlining basic metabolic pathways.

I nearly left it at that, but my eagle-eyed colleague Mike Perry pointed out to me that I had undertaken, in the diagram on β oxidation in the first edition, to write a song about the fate of odd-number carbon chain fatty acids, in the event that there was ever a second edition. So I took pen and paper upstairs on the 85 bus from Roehampton to Putney Bridge station. Owing to extensive road works it was a slow journey, and the song was completed in one go. Mike then exercised his gentle charm to give a very strong hint about the centrality of ketone bodies in intermediary metabolism. Fortunately, Putney Bridge was still a traffic jam the following day. I don't imagine that we'll make a cassette of the new songs, but the tunes are pretty well known – two from Gilbert and Sullivan, two old American folksongs, a popular hymn (and Welsh rugby song) and a Christmas carol. Apologies to my friends in Nagoya and elsewhere who don't know them – but they're easy to pick out on the piano with the music provided. Happy singing, and good luck in trying to make the verses scan!

FOREWORD

Life with biochemistry—indeed with all sciences—is not always as solemn as the textbooks and scientific periodicals suggest. From 1923 to 1931 the Cambridge Biochemical Laboratory, at that time under Sir Frederick Gowland Hopkins, one of the world's foremost centres of biochemistry, published once a year a highly original and amusing house journal called *Brighter Biochemistry*.

It was written by the members of the laboratory, including Hopkins, J. B. S. Haldane and other distinguished scientists. It covered those features of biochemistry which, though not acceptable for publication to the Editor of the *Biochemical Journal*, were nevertheless part of life with biochemistry. *Brighter Biochemistry* reported, and commented on, all sorts of goings-on in the laboratory. It made delightful reading then, and still does so today—some fifty years after it was produced.

Some verses by J. B. S. Haldane give a flavour of *Brighter Biochemistry*. He wrote an imaginary 'Annual Report' to the Secretary of the Sir William Dunn Trustees (benefactors of the Laboratory). The 150 line 'report' begins by describing a class experiment in which some students were successful in preparing tryptophan from casein, while others were not:

> Sir, on the upper floor the classes
> Included genii and asses,
> The former got out tryptophane,
> The latter poured it down the drain.

He further muses on the fact that animals cannot carry out photosynthesis:

> I cannot synthesise a bun
> By simply sitting in the sun.

xi

Some nasty smells inspired him to these rhymes:

> I must admit I always flee
> When offered drinks of NH_3 ;
> I fear that $NaNO_2$
> Would turn my haemoglobin blue.

The number of copies of *Brighter Biochemistry* was, of course, small. The surviving ones now have a considerable collectors' value. Each edition of *Brighter Biochemistry* was eagerly awaited and avidly read and I therefore feel confident that Professor Baum's contribution to the brighter side of biochemistry will be welcomed widely. The songs are skilful, witty and amusing. They may even help the student to get over examination hurdles; they certainly will give much pleasure.

Sir Hans Krebs

CONTENTS

THE MICHAELIS ANTHEM
(Tune: "The Red Flag")

The substrate changed, by an enzyme,
Initially, in unit time,
Varies, (if not in excess),
With substrate concentration, $[S]$.
If enzyme concentration's low,
And reaction back from product's slow,
Then, if we choose a steady-state,
Velocity and $[S]$ relate.

This relationship can be derived
As Briggs and Haldane first contrived:
The unbound enzyme, $[E]$, we guess
Is $[E_O]$ (total), less $[ES]$.
$k_1 [S] [E]$ gives $[ES]$ formation
And $k_2 [ES]$, dissociation
And $[ES]$ gives the product, P,
At a rate that's $[ES]$ times k_3.

When $[ES]$ is at the steady-state
These terms are all seen to relate
$([E_O]$ *less* $[ES]) . k_1 [S]$
Equals $(k_2 + k_3)[ES]$.
Now the maximum velocity
Is $k_3 [E_O]$, (or big V).
These terms can be manipulated
If one more definition's stated.

Define as K_m (just for fun)
$(k_2 + k_3)$ on k_1
And note that v (velocity),
Is always $[ES]$ times k_3.
Then rearranging these relations
We get the final rate equation:
V times $[S]$ on $K_m + [S]$
Is v (initial) — more or less.

THE RED FLAG

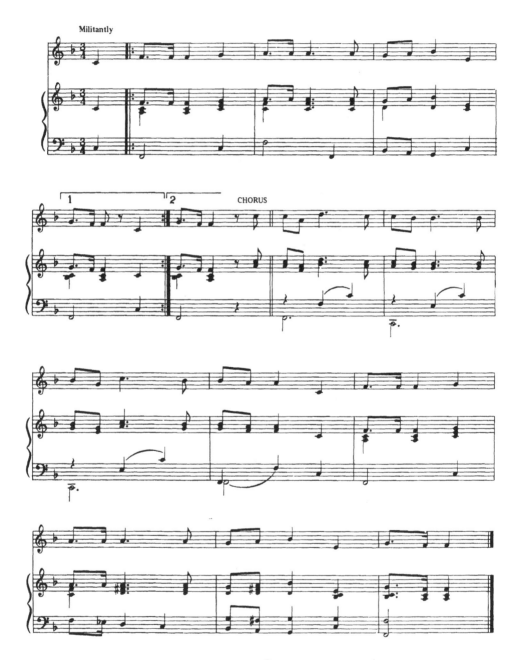

Enzyme Kinetics

The formation of product P from substrate S catalysed by enzyme E, via the enzyme-substrate complex ES, can be represented by the equation:

$$E + S \underset{k_2}{\overset{k_1}{\rightleftharpoons}} ES \xrightarrow{k_3} E + P$$

The relationship between the concentration of S and the initial rate of product formation can be derived, assuming that the concentration of enzyme is low compared to that of substrate (so that ES formation does not significantly alter the concentration of S), and that reaction back from P is initially negligible.

Let total enzyme concentration be $[Eo]$ and concentration of free enzyme be $[E]$.

Then $[E] = [Eo] - [ES]$ (i)

Rate of formation of $ES = k_1[E][S]$ (ii)

Rate of dissociation of $ES = k_2[ES]$ (iii)

Rate of product formation $= k_3[ES]$ (iv)

When the concentration of ES has reached a steady state

$$k_1[E][S] = k_2[ES] + k_3[ES] \tag{v}$$

Substituting from equation (i)

$$k_1[S]([Eo] - [ES]) = (k_2 + k_3)[ES] \tag{vi}$$

Now velocity (i.e. rate of product formation)

$$v = k_3[ES] \tag{iv}$$

$$\therefore [ES] = \frac{v}{k_3} \tag{vii}$$

The maximum velocity (V) when all the enzyme is saturated with substrate, i.e. when $[ES] = [Eo]$ is $k_3[Eo]$ (viii)

$$\therefore [Eo] = \frac{V}{k_3} \tag{ix}$$

Substituting (vii) and (ix) in (vi)

$$k_1[S] \frac{(V - v)}{k_3} = (k_2 + k_3) \frac{v}{k_3} \tag{x}$$

Multiply both sides by k_3/k_1

$$[S](V - v) = \left(\frac{k_2 + k_3}{k_1} \right) v \tag{xi}$$

$$\therefore [S]V = \left(\frac{k_2 + k_3}{k_1} + [S] \right) v \tag{xii}$$

Define $\frac{k_2 + k_3}{k_1}$ as K_m (the Michaelis constant)

Divide both sides by $K_m + [S]$

Then v (initial rate) $= \dfrac{V[S]}{K_m + [S]}$ (xiii)

(Note that when $K_m = [S]$, $v = V/2$, i.e. K_m = substrate concentration for half maximal velocity.)

3

IN PRAISE OF E.M.P.
(Tune: "The British Grenadiers")

Some pathways lead to glory, like Hatch and Slack and Knoop,
Utter, Calvin, Cori—a most distinguished group,
But of all of nature's pathways, we sing the praise today
Of Parnas, Embden, Meyerhof—the glycolytic way.

Glucose, by hexokinase is turned to G6P
(You might use glucokinase, you must use ATP)
And, note, glycogenolysis (when stores are in the cell)
Gives G1P which then mutates to G6P as well.

The moiety of glucose, in the succeeding phase
Is transferred to a ketose by an isomerase
Phosphofructokinase now, acts on that F6P;
Fructose 1-6 bisphosphate is the product that's set free.

The kinase is effected quite complicatedly
And as you'll have suspected it uses ATP;
FDP by aldolase is split reversibly
To phosphoglyceraldehyde, also DHAP.

The former and the latter can each equilibrate—
It really doesn't matter for metabolic fate—
So follow PG aldehyde and double what you see,
You'll get the total balance sheet for a hexose moiety.

There's now a novel facet, for NAD's reduced
But carboxylic acid is not what is produced,
ΔE's substantial, and energy's conserved
(For otherwise the pathway would, quite frankly, be absurd).

The complex oxidation of PG aldehyde
Gives by phosphorylation an acid anhydride,
And that diphosphoglycerate reacts with ADP
The kinase making ATP, of course reversibly.

. . . / . . .

The product's composition, 3-phosphoglycerate
From 3 to 2 position can readily mutate
And now 2-phosphoglycerate does something rather strange—
Electrons on C 2 and 3 proceed to rearrange.

Thus, redox-dehydration, catalysed by enolase
Gives P.E.P. formation and bond energy raise
So phospho-enol pyruvate reacts with ADP
The kinase making ATP, but *not* reversibly.

In anaerobiosis, pyruvate's not the end;
The problem we suppose is not hard to comprehend;
The dehydrogenation to phosphoglycerate
Would grind to halt if NAD could not regenerate.

The answer is quite subtle, pyruvate is reduced,
Instead of malate shuttle, L-lactate is produced;
Lactate dehydrogenase performs that noble feat,
NADH is oxidised; the pathway is complete.

The balance sheet you'll see shows transfer of energy,
Two ATPs from glucose, and three from G1P.
That's good, but oh to use the way where pyruvate's reduced
With decarboxylation first, then ethanol produced!

THE BRITISH GRENADIERS

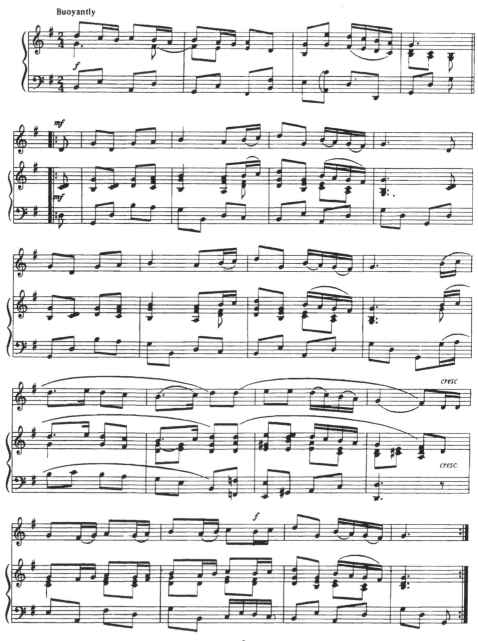

6

Glycolysis

[glycogen] $\xrightarrow{1}$ glucose-1-phosphate

P_i

glucose

glucose-6-phosphate

ATP → ADP, 2

3

CH_2OH ... OPO_3^{2-}

$CH_2OPO_3^{2-}$

4

$^{2-}O_3POCH_2$ ... CH_2OH

fructose-6-phosphate

5, ATP → ADP

$^{2-}O_3POCH_2$ ... $CH_2OPO_3^{2-}$

fructose-1,6 bisphosphate

6
7

$\begin{array}{l} CHO \\ H-C-OH \\ CH_2OPO_3^{2-} \end{array}$
D-glyceraldehyde-3-phosphate

$\begin{array}{l} CH_2OPO_3^{2-} \\ C=O \\ CH_2OH \end{array}$
dihydroxyacetone phosphate

$\begin{array}{l} COO^- \\ H-C-OH \\ CH_3 \end{array}$
2(lactate)

$\begin{array}{l} CH_2OH \\ CH_3 \end{array}$
2(ethanol)

P_i, 8, NAD$^+$ (X 2) → NADH + H$^+$ ········→ NADH + H$^+$ ← NAD$^+$ (X 2) | 13 ← ← NAD$^+$ (X 2) | 15 → NADH + H$^+$)

$\begin{array}{l} O \\ \| \\ C-OPO_3^{2-} \\ H-C-OH \\ CH_2OPO_3^{2-} \end{array}$
2(1,3-diphosphoglycerate)

$\begin{array}{l} COO^- \\ C=O \\ CH_3 \end{array}$
2(pyruvate)

(X 2) 14, CO_2

$\begin{array}{l} CHO \\ CH_3 \end{array}$
2(acetaldehyde)

9 (X 2), ADP → ATP

(X 2) 12, ATP → ADP

$\begin{array}{l} COO^- \\ H-C-OH \\ CH_2OPO_3^{2-} \end{array}$
2(3-phosphoglycerate)

$\begin{array}{l} COO^- \\ C-OPO_3^{2-} \\ \| \\ CH_2 \end{array}$
2(phosphoenolpyruvate)

10 (X 2)

$\begin{array}{l} COO^- \\ H-C-OPO_3^{2-} \\ CH_2OH \end{array}$
2(2-phosphoglycerate)

11 (X 2), H_2O

Enzymes:
1. glycogen phosphorylase
2. glucokinase and hexokinase
3. phosphoglucomutase
4. phosphoglucoisomerase
5. phosphofructokinase
6. aldolase
7. triose phosphate isomerase
8. phosphoglyceraldehyde dehydrogenase
9. phosphoglyceric acid kinase
10. phosphoglyceromutase
11. enolase
12. pyruvate kinase
13. lactate dehydrogenase
14. pyruvate decarboxylase }
15. alcohol dehydrogenase } (alcohol formation in, say, yeast)

7

WALTZ ROUND THE CYCLE
(Tune: "Waltzing Matilda")

Once a jolly pyruvate enters the matrix
Of a mitochondrion, so they say,
A decarboxylating, complex dehydrogenase
Converts it to acetyl co-enzyme A.

Waltz round the cycle
Waltz round the cycle
Waltz round the TCA cycle today.
A decarboxylating, complex dehydrogenase
Turns pyruvate to acetyl CoA.

Oxaloacetate looking for a partner
Thinks "active acetate" looks OK;
Condensing enzyme arranging a merger
Makes a new citrate, and kicks out CoA.

Waltz round the cycle
Waltz round the cycle
Waltz round the TCA cycle today.
Condensing enzyme arranging a merger
Makes a new citrate, and kicks out CoA.

Along comes aconitase, a hydro-dehydratase,
Gives isocitrate reversibiy.
Then its dehydrogenase gives NADH,
Carbon dioxide and α-OG.

Waltz round the cycle
Waltz round the cycle
Waltz round the TCA cycle with me.
Then its dehydrogenase gives NADH,
Carbon dioxide and α-OG.

. . . / . . .

Off with the CO_2. Another oxidation
Just like the PDC previously.
Succinyl CoA with a thiokinase
Yields succinate and GTP.

Waltz round the cycle
Waltz round the cycle
Waltz round the TCA cycle with me.
Succinyl CoA with a thiokinase
Yields succinate and GTP.

Succinate's oxidised by its dehydrogenase
Reducing FAD, giving fumarate;
Fumarase makes malate; another dehydrogenase
Generates oxaloacetate.

Waltz round the cycle
Waltz round the cycle
Waltz round the TCA cycle, mate.
Fumarase makes malate; another dehydrogenase
Generates oxaloacetate.

Abbreviations: TCA   tricarboxylic acid
α-OG   α-oxoglutarate
PDC   pyruvate dehydrogenase complex

WALTZING MATILDA

MARIE COWEN

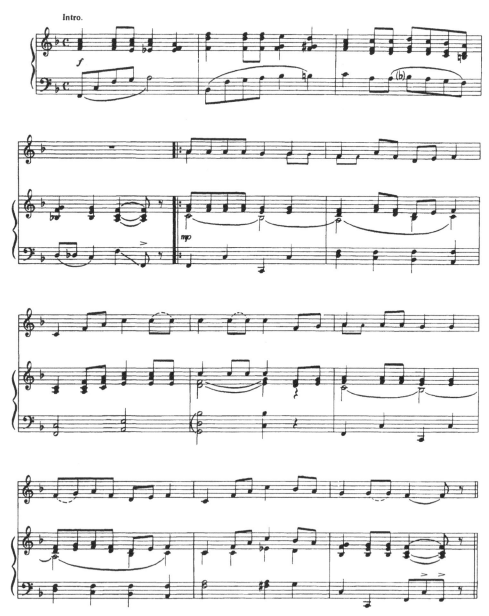

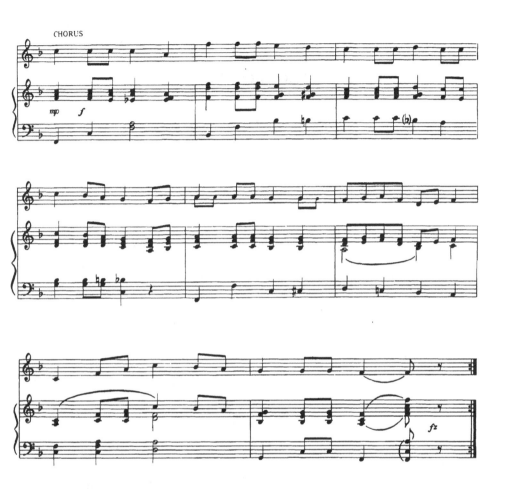

11

CITRIC ACID CYCLE
(Tricarboxylic acid cycle, Krebs' cycle)

$$CH_3 - \overset{O}{\overset{\|}{C}} - COO^-$$
pyruvate

CoASH — NAD$^+$

CO_2 → NADH

$$CH_3\overset{O}{\overset{\|}{C}} - SCoA$$
acetyl-SCoA

H_2O (1) CoASH

$^-OOCCH_2CCOO^-$
oxaloacetate

NAD$^+$ (8) NADH

H

$^-OOCCH_2 - \overset{H}{\underset{OH}{C}} - COO^-$
L-malate

(7)

H_2O

H

$OOCC = CCOO^-$
H
fumarate

FADH$_2$

(6)

FAD

$^-OOCCH_2CH_2COO^-$
succinate

GTP

(5)

CoASH   GDP

P$_i$

$^-OOCCH_2CH_2\overset{O}{\overset{\|}{C}}-SCoA$
succinyl-SCoA

CO_2

NADH (4) NAD$^+$

CoASH

^-OOC, H C
^-OOC CH$_2$COO
cis-aconitate

$-H_2O$

(remains bound to enzyme)

$+H_2O$

isomerization

$$\begin{array}{c} COO^- \\ CH_2 \\ HO-C-COO^- \\ CH_2 \\ COO^- \end{array}$$
citrate

(2)

$$\begin{array}{c} COO^- \\ H-C-OH \\ ^-OOC-C-H \\ CH_2 \\ COO^- \end{array}$$
isocitrate

NAD$^+$

(3) Mg^{2+}

NADH — CO$_2$

$$\begin{array}{c} COO^- \\ C=O \\ CH_2 \\ CH_2 \\ COO^- \end{array}$$
α-oxoglutarate

1. citrate-condensing enzyme
2. aconitase
3. isocitrate dehydrogenase
4. α-oxoglutarate dehydrogenase
5. succinate thiokinase
6. succinate dehydrogenase
7. fumarase
8. L-malate dehydrogenase

β OXIDATION

(Tune: "There is a Tavern in the Town")

There is a pathway in the cell (in the cell)
That metabolises well (awfully well)
Fatty acyl chains in a most effective way
To acetyl coenzyme A.
It's called β oxidation, and by way of explanation
In the mitochondrial matrix is the major part.
It starts however on the cytosolic side
With fatty acids coming from triglyceride
Activated in the thiokinase way
To thioester of CoA.

Acyl CoA can't permeate (permeate)
The inner membrane to its fate (sad to state)
But a transferase now comes upon the scene
Making fatty acyl carnitine.
And there now is permeation, and a new transacylation
Generating acyl CoA in the matrix space.
We now begin upon an oxidation phase
With FAD-dependent dehydrogenase
(The flavoprotein is oxidised again
By ETF, thence by the chain).

Of two H atoms thus relieved (thus relieved)
Desaturation's been achieved (been achieved)
And as they came from the α:β slot
Enoyl CoA's what we've got.
And it's in that same position we get aqueous addition
That is catalysed by enoyl hydratase
OH addition's onto carbon number 3
. (Creating thus a centre of asymmetry)
Giving β hydroxy acyl CoA
Which now proceeds upon its way.

. . . / . . .

Keto formation next we see (next we see)
From β-ol plus NAD (NAD)
The hydroxyacyl dehydrogenase
Prepares the way for thiolase
And, say, who would be a critic, of a cleavage thiolytic
Of a simple β keto thioester bond?
Coenzyme A is the attacking moiety
And acetyl CoA the product that's set free,
So the common feature each such sequence shares
Is stripping carbons off in pairs.

An acyl CoA thus is left (thus is left)
Of two-carbon fragment bereft (oh, bereft!)
Ready activated for another round
All citric acid cycle bound.
And if you perchance enquire, I'll simply point out that that spiral
Has analogies to steps starting from succinate.*
Each turn of its can give you five times ATP
Apart from acetyl CoA that is set free.
Activation puts two squiggles up the spout
But just you think what you get out!

*If this is not immediately apparent to you, just think about it!

THERE IS A TAVERN IN THE TOWN

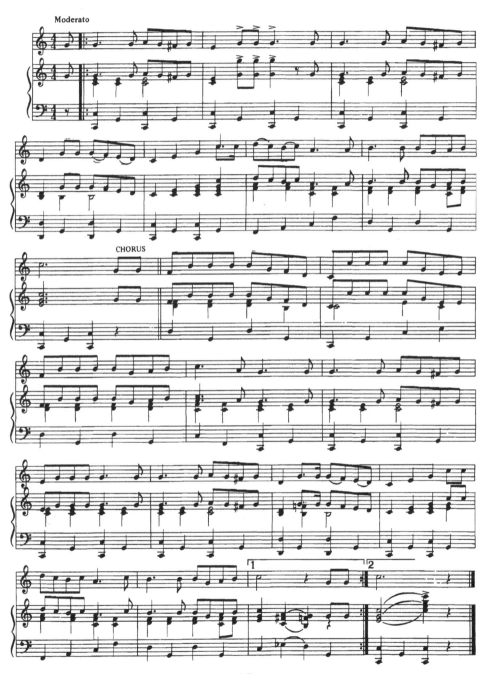

Fatty Acid Oxidation

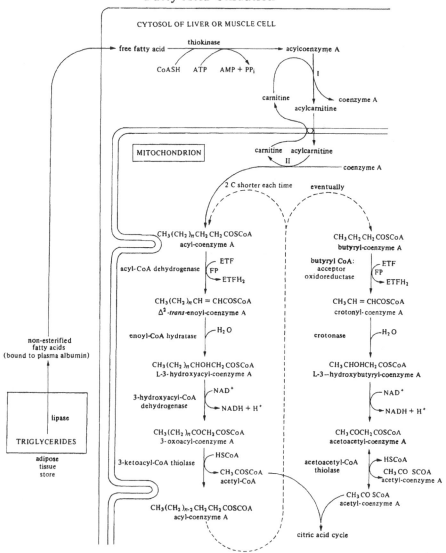

I and II are membrane-associated carnityl transferases
ETF = electron transferring flavoprotein
FP = flavoprotein

Notes: –   (i) C3 on the diagram is equivalent to the β C in the song
               (ii) ETFH$_2$ and NADH are reoxidised by the respiratory chain.
               (iii) Fatty acids with an odd number of carbon atoms ultimately yield one molecule of propionyl CoA.
                    Perhaps in the next edition I will write a song about how this is then metabolised.

Note in 2nd edition: I've kept my promise! See page 70.

THE BATTLE HYMN OF THE AEROBES
(Tune: "The Battle Hymn of the Republic")

Mine eyes have seen the glory of respiratory chains
In every mitochondrion, intrinsic to membranes,
Functionally organised in complex sub-domains
Where electrons flow along.
Glory, glory, respiration! *(three times)*
Where electrons flow along.

Each chain is a mosaic of Complexes I to IV
Embedded in the lipid (which is what the lipid's for)
But that is not sufficient, there are *two* components more
Where electrons, *etc.*

The first is a small cytochrome that rolls around the place
That's easily extractable from cytoplasmic face
That restores respiration if you just add back a trace,
Where electrons, *etc.*

The other's a benzoquinone that is ubiquitous,
It floats around the lipid phase with hardly any fuss,
For mobile pooling function it's become synonymous,
Where electrons, *etc.*

NADH to CoQ_{10}'s the job of Complex I,
It contains a single flavin—(and FMN is the one)
And all that non-haem iron can't *just* be there for fun,
Where electrons, *etc.*

Succinate is oxidised by way of Complex II,
It starts off with FAD and it reduces Q,
And just to make it complex it's got non-haem iron too,
Where electrons, *etc.*

From CoQ through to cyto. c requires Complex III,
It's got c_1 and iron too and two species of b,
There's an antimycin-binding site, core-proteins two or three,
Where electrons, *etc.*

. . . / . . .

17

Finally to Complex IV where oxygen's reduced,
Two coppers, a and a_3 (which in yeast can be induced),
Fine end to the finest chain that Nature has produced,
Where electrons, *etc.*

(Most of the information in the above song derives from work carried out in the laboratories of David E. Green in Madison, Wisconsin. To David, my friend and mentor, this song is therefore dedicated.)

BATTLE HYMN OF THE REPUBLIC

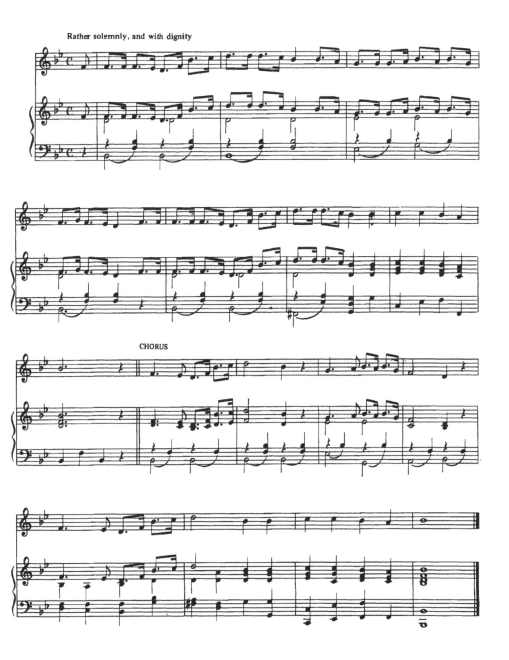

The Respiratory Chain

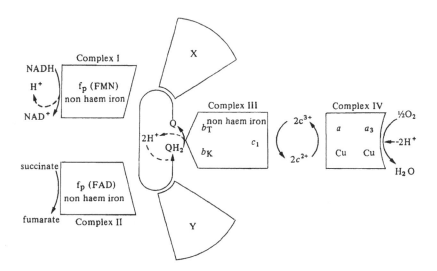

X and Y are other ubiquinone-reducing flavoproteins (eg. from α glycerophosphate cr fatty acyl coenzyme A).

NB.   (i) The diagram illustrates functional, not structural inter-relationships.

           (ii) All complexes are intrinsic to the inner mitochondrial membrane.

           (iii) c (cytochrome c) is located extrinsically to the cytosol-facing surface.

           (iv) Q (ubiquinone$_{10}$) is relatively mobile within the hydrophobic regions of the membrane, but may in part be functionally compartmentalised between protein-associated sub-pools.

THE CHEMIOSMOTIC THEORY

(Tune: "The Eton Boating Song")

Oxidative phosphorylation, exceedingly hard to explain,
Accounting for cation movement and why you need a membrane,
But the chemiosmotic theory gives membranous structure a role,
Accounts for uncoupler action and respiratory control.

Mitochondrial inner membranes have redox complexes inlaid
And their topological features direct a proton cascade,
Electrons and protons in symport move outward on enzymic track
Followed by charge separation as electrons alone cross back.

In the simplest of formulations all reductions on matrical side
Need protons as well as electrons (hydrogen atoms implied)
Whilst reductions at external surface (for example of cytochrome *c*)
Take electrons alone to pass inwards leaving protonic charges free.

Now the net result of this looping (for succinate, say, you loop twice)
Makes coupled respiratory complex charge-separating device
And the driving force for this process is potential change (ΔE),
Redox energy thus converted is transduced to proticity.

Now, control upon respiration, and more separation of charge
Is imposed as membrane potential becomes increasingly large,
But uniport cation uptake on porter or ionophore
Starts to collapse the potential, permits respiration once more.

Such uptake is somewhat restricted, by internal buffering state,
As more protons are ejected, so ΔpH gets great,
And the motive force of the protons which slows respiration when high
Is a term with ΔpH in, plus membrane potential (or ψ).

As ψ drives cation uptake and ΔpH becomes great
An antiport P_i:hydroxyl can make salts accumulate,
But a far more important process that's linked to this proticity
Is of course hydro-dehydration between P_i and ADP.

. . . / . . .

For inlaid across that same membrane is Fo with protonic well
F_1-ATPase stuck on it (by OSCP they tell)
When ATP's split in that headpiece, protons come from the matrix side,
The rest of the reaction water, coming in as C-side oxide.

So that whole ATPase complex is a proton pumping device,
At high p.m.f.* it reverses, which is really rather nice;
Not only will ATP breakdown take up ions reversibly,
But p.m.f. from respiration drives the making of ATP.

So to summarise we've a membrane, proton impermeable too,
With proticity generators, conveniently plugged through;
Each thus interacts with the other, 'squiggle's' just p.m.f. and no more,
An uncoupler simply functions by acting as protonophore.

*Proton motive force; but think of it as Peter Mitchell formulation.

THE ETON BOATING SONG

Original words by
William Cory Johnson

Music by
Algernon Drummond & Evelyn Wodehouse

Allegro con spirito *(Tempo di Barcarola)*

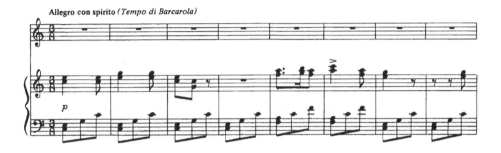

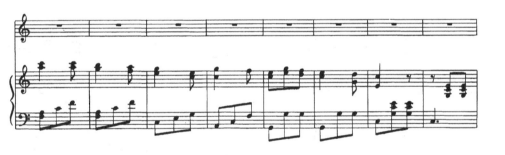

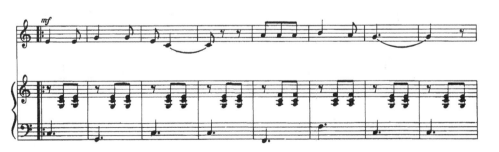

23

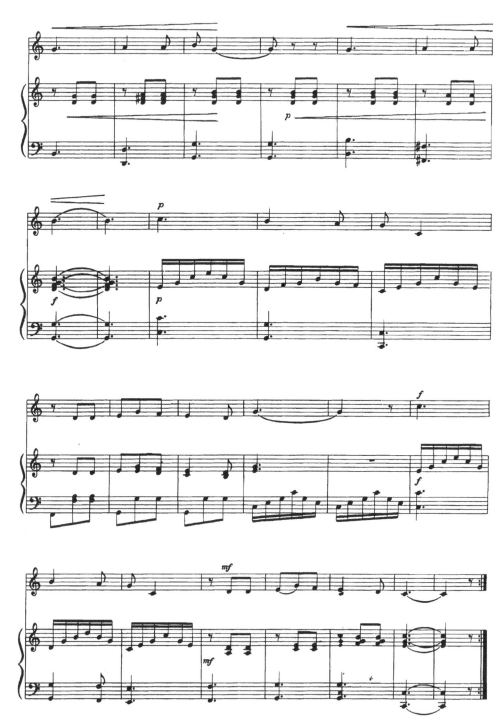

24

Chemiosmotic Theory

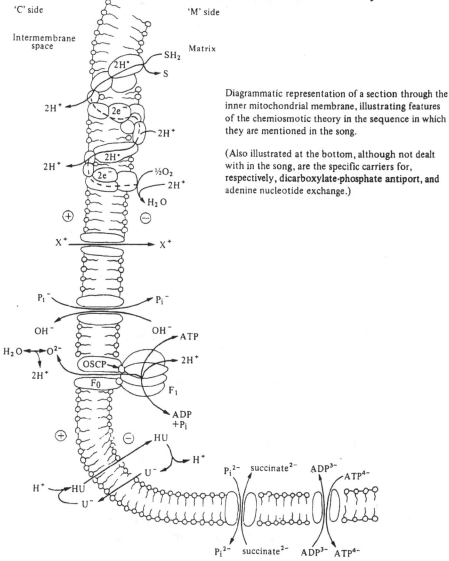

Diagrammatic representation of a section through the inner mitochondrial membrane, illustrating features of the chemiosmotic theory in the sequence in which they are mentioned in the song.

(Also illustrated at the bottom, although not dealt with in the song, are the specific carriers for, respectively, dicarboxylate-phosphate antiport, and adenine nucleotide exchange.)

Note in 2nd edition:

This diagram, which matches the words in the song, is now somewhat outdated. Observed stoichiometries of proton extrusion are inconsistent with the simple loop formulation. It is now thought that around 4, 4 and 2 protons are pumped out per pair of electrons transversing, respectively, Complexes I, III and IV, (see *The Battle Hymn of the Aerobes*). Detailed mechanisms for Complexes I and IV are still controversial; in Complex III, the 'Q cycle' probably operates, which is an elaboration of the loop concept. Also the ATP-synthase mechanism is now thought not to be as illustrated here. ATP is believed to form spontaneously in the F_1 sector, but is then too tightly bound to be released. The energy made available by the return of $3H^+$ via the F_0 sector is then somehow transduced into releasing the ATP. Export of ATP^{4-} in exchange for ATP^{3-} (see diagram) effectively 'costs' a further H^+. These protonic stoichiometries suggest P/O ratios of 1.5 and 2.5 for the oxidation, respectively, of succinate and NADH.

25

PHOTOSYNTHESIS
(Tune: "Auld Lang Syne")

When sunlight bathes the chloroplast, and photons are absorbed
The energy's transduced so fast that food is quickly stored,
Photosynthetic greenery traps light the spectrum through
Then dark pathway machinery fixes the CO_2.

Two chlorophylls (a, b to you) are cleverly deployed
In photosystems I and II, within the thylakoid
System I takes energy, at 700 (red)
While system II (with pigment b) takes 680 instead.

At manganese on centre II, see oxygen displace
As water's split, and protons too, leave membrane inner face
Electrons that we thus produce, cross, 'photo-fortified'
Plastoquinone then to reduce, upon the other side.

Meanwhile at I, chlorophyll a is photo-oxidised
(At 'positive holes', formed that way, electrons are much prized),
Electrons that we thus eject reduce NADP
With ferredoxin we suspect, as intermediary.

That hole in I we now negate, plastoquinol moves in
With b and f to mediate, and plastocyanin,
That redox loop, potential large, runs exergonically
With membrane-separated charge, and thence to ATP.

That Z track by electron pair, reduced NADP,
Plucked oxygen from water's care, and made some ATP.
Now we've got power to reduce, and ATP to spare,
Food in the dark we can produce, from CO_2 in air.

Ribulose diphosphate takes, a mole of CO_2
Gives two 3-phosphoglycerates, (if Calvin's story's true)
NADPH now provides, reducing power to make
Two phosphoglyceraldehydes (as ATP we break).

. . . / . . .

26

There now occurs a jolly jig (the details we'll ignore)
With carbon chains both small and big, to ribulose once more,
Each time round, as CO_2, is fixed we've chains to spare
And we can make hexoses new, from triose phosphate pair.

Other routes involve C_4, or pyruvate to fat,
NADPH as before, is vital still for that,
ATP still provides the drive, the moral still is this—
The one thing that keeps life alive is photosynthesis.

AULD LANG SYNE

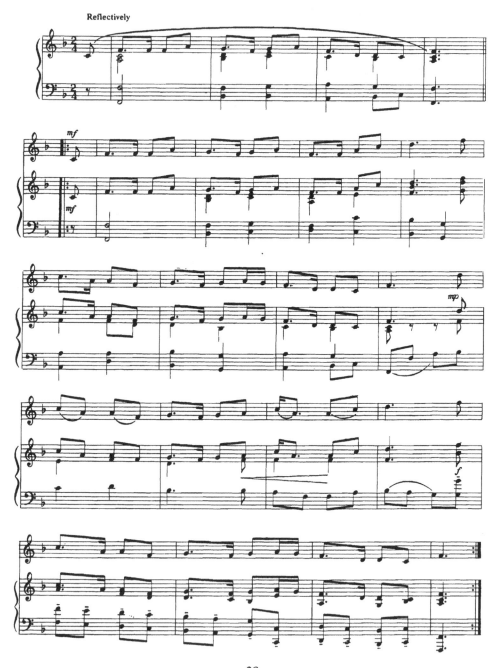

Photosynthesis

A. Light Reactions

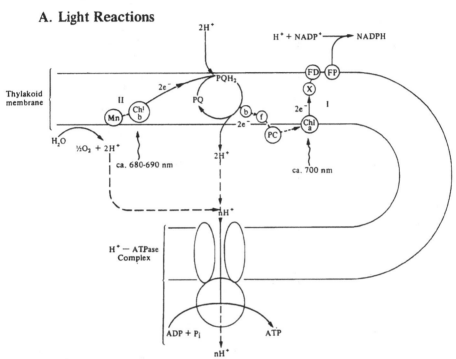

NB.   (i) The precise sequence and stoichiometries are speculative.
        (ii) The chlorophylls designated are not exclusive to their respective reaction centres.

PQ = plastoquinone, FD = Ferredoxin, FP = flavoprotein, PC = Plastocyanin, b & f = cytochromes

B. Dark Reactions

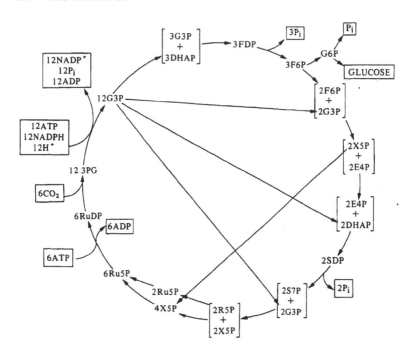

Diagrammatic summary of the Calvin cycle.

Note that six ribulose diphosphates (RuDP) combine with six CO_2 to yield twelve 3-phosphoglycerates (3PG). Two of these give rise to glucose; the other ten eventually regenerate six RuDP to continue the fixation process.

(The Hatch-Slack C_4 pathway, alluded to briefly in the song, might be dealt with separately in the next edition, if there is a demand for it).

Key:

3PG = 3-phosphoglyceric acid
G3P = glyceraldehyde 3-phosphate
DHAP = dihydroxyacetone phosphate
FDP = fructose 1,6-diphosphate
F6P = fructose 6-phosphate
G6P = glucose 6-phosphate
E4P = erythrose 4-phosphate
X5P = xylulose 5-phosphate
SDP = sedoheptulose 1,7-diphosphate
S7P = sedoheptulose 7-phosphate
R5P = ribose 5-phosphate
Ru5P = ribulose 5-phosphate
RuDP = ribulose 1,5-diphosphate

30

BLOOD SUGAR
(Tune: "The Road to the Isles")

If you've not eaten and the glucose in your blood
Begins to fall to levels rather low
You start off processes that nip right in the bud
That crisis, by the paths we'll shortly show.

When a hormone hits receptors on the surface of a cell
(A hormone such as glucagon's implied)
Then an enzyme's activated in that cell membrane as well
Albeit on the cytosolic side.

That cyclase enzyme then can act on ATP
Making second messenger quite easily,
A cyclic diester that acts allosterically
Sets protein kinase active centre free.

Then that kinase starts a cascade of enzyme activity
By phosphorylation altering their style
So the synthetase for glycogen can change from a to b
And slow synthetic action for a while.

Liver phosphorylase, phosphorylated whole,
The form in which activity is great,
Now expresses its phosphorylysing role
And mobilizes stored carbohydrate.

So now non-reducing glucosyls are plucked from glycogen
With P_i yielding lots of G.1.P.
(And of course there's a debranching step just every now and then)
But how is glucose now to be set free?

Mutating G.1.P. gives rise to G.6.P,
Glucose-6-phosphatase now acts as well
In hepatocyte e.r. bound intrinsically
Releases unbound glucose from the cell.

. . . / . . .

But when you've run out of glycogen that pathway has to end
And you've got to make your sugars *de novo*
And if you've got C_4 moieties or C_3 to extend
To gluconeogenesis you'll go.

As starting material lactate, say, would do,
Or alanine if you transaminate,
Cycle intermediates are quite useful too
Since all can give oxaloacetate.

For the first two lead to pyruvate, you can carboxylate
Utilizing CO_2 and ATP
Then PEP carboxykinase on oxaloacetate
Completes the clever shunt to P.E.P.

Once you've P.E.P. available you're close to victory,
You just reverse the glycolytic phase,
The small embarrassment at F 1-6 *bis* P
Is by-passed by a single phosphatase.

And so once again you'll find yourself with loads of G.6.P.
(Though it cost you ATP I rather fear)
And when your liver's phosphatase sets all that glucose free
Hypoglycaemic symptoms disappear.

Publisher's note

Unfortunately, it has not been possible for us to reproduce the music for "The Road to the Isles" due to copyright problems. However, anyone interested in obtaining it should write to the publisher, Boosey & Hawkes Ltd., 295 Regent Street, London W1R 8JH.

Maintenance of Blood Glucose

A. Glycogenolysis

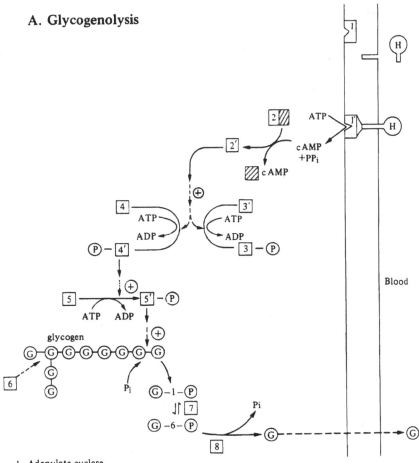

1 Adenylate cyclase
2 Protein kinase
3 Glycogen synthetase
4 Phosphorylase kinase
5 Phosphorylase
6 Debranching enzyme system
7 Phosphoglucomutase
8 Glucose-6-phosphatase

$\xrightarrow{\oplus}$ Site of action of active form of enzyme ($\boxed{x'}$) at next step in cascade.

$\boxed{x}$, $\boxed{x'}$ Inactive and active forms, respectively, of enzymes affected in the cascade.

33

B. Gluconeogenesis

(from lactate as an example)

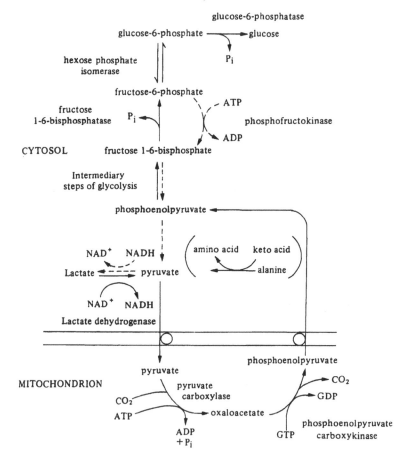

NB. 2 lactate molecules (and hence 2 molecules of phosphoenol pyruvate)
are required for the synthesis of one hexose molecule.

- - ► = direction of glycolytic pathway. Also, note that the location of PEP
carboxykinase (and hence the nature of transport steps required)
varies between species.

C. G-protein as link between glucagon-receptor and adenylate cyclase

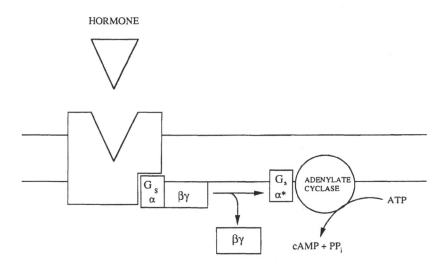

The song, and diagram A, imply direct interaction between hormone-receptor complex and cyclase. In fact, binding of glucagon indirectly affects the G_s (s, for stimulatory) protein that is associated with the cytoplasmic side of the receptor, leading to replacement of bound GDP by GTP. This alters the conformation of the α sub-unit, leading to dissociation from it of the β and γ sub-units, allowing the α sub-unit – GTP complex ($G_s\ \alpha^*$) to leave the receptor and translocate along the membrane to bind to and activate the cyclase.

THE GLYOXYLATE CYCLE
(Tune: "The Lincolnshire Poacher"*)

All mammals are superior we confidently state,
But there are some criteria by which we're second rate,
For *our* anaplerotic routes can't make glyoxylate
And so we fall flat at turning of fat
Into new carbohydrate.

For gluconeogenesis we must make P.E.P.
And PEP carboxykinase turns C_4 into C_3
But oxaloacetic can't be made so easily
(Acetyl CoA in the TCA
Ends as CO_2 set free).

But humble *Tetrahymena* or leaf or oily seed
Can manifest a pathway that is elegant indeed,
Two new enzyme activities equip them to succeed
At turning with style all spare acetyl
To the sugars that they need.

The pathway's compartmentalised 'twixt metabolic homes
Involving mitochondria and the peroxisomes
(The microbodies otherwise or else glyoxisomes)
But first we must start with the mito part
As fat oxidative zones.

For β oxidation there yields *acetyl CoA*
Which joins *oxaloacetate* the condensation way,
And isocitrate soon can leave, exchanged for malate, say,
(But citrate as well, as we'll shortly tell
Has an export role to play).

Isocitrate meets one enzyme we've not met before,
A lyase that can split C_6 to C_2 plus C_4
Glyoxalate plus *succinate*, of latter we'll hear more,
But glyoxylate has a novel fate
That firstly we shall explore.

. . . / . . .

We're β oxidising so we've *acetyl CoA*
(Exported from the mitos in the form of citrate, say,
The C_4 from the cleavage going back the other way)
And now is the time for a new enzyme
Its synthetic part to play.

The enzyme's malate synthase, and that's just what it can do,
Glyoxylate plus acetyl is simply two plus two,
The product is thus *malate* and it should be clear to you
That we've now achieved what we said we need,
An anaplerotic coup.

The whole reaction balance sheet we now can simply state,
Two acetyls have entered plus oxaloacetate,
The product is one malate and a mole of succinate,
So we've more C_4 than we had before
Which is cause to celebrate.

The C_4 acids give rise in the usual kind of way
To oxaloacetic (by the citric cycle, say)
Which can keep the pool increasing with more acetyl CoA
Or give—oh bliss—net synthesis
Of glucose—shout hurray!

*The repeated rhyming of "way" with "say" (and often with "play") is an old Lincolnshire tradition. The additional rhyme with "CoA" is, of course, of more recent origin.

THE LINCOLNSHIRE POACHER

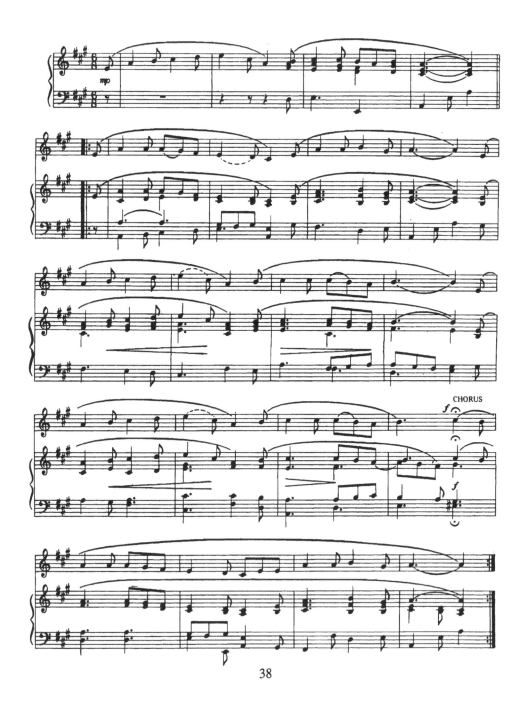

CHORUS

The Glyoxylate cycle

(NB the exact mode of compartmentation varies between species)

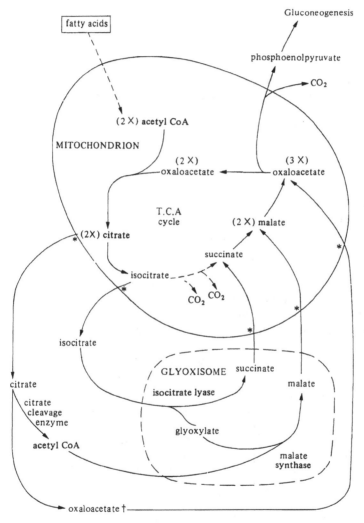

Net result: 2 Acetyl CoA + 2 oxaloacetate $\longrightarrow$ 3 oxaloacetate $\longrightarrow$ 2 oxaloacetate + PEP + CO_2
$\equiv$ 2 Acetyl CoA $\longrightarrow$ PEP + CO_2
(* specific exchange diffusion carriers)
(† may be reduced in the cytosol to malate before re-entering the mitochondrion)

THE PENTOSE PHOSPHATE SHUNT
(Tune: "Macnamara's Band")

If you're converting carbohydrate into triglycerides,
If you need pentose moieties to make nucleotides,
You'll find that Embden-Meyerhof is not the game to play
And you'll do your biosynthesis the pentose phosphate way.

Chorus: With transaldolase, transketolase, G6PDH too,
             Six times six gives fives times six plus six of CO_2
             Carbons passing to and fro, the back becomes the front,
             Did you ever see a pathway like the pentose phosphate shunt?

First G6P is oxidised, NADP reduced
To give gluconolactone (as might well have been deduced).
The lactone is then hydrolysed to make the gluconate
And decarboxylation is its metabolic fate.

There ends the oxidative phase, now multiply by three,
An intermediary balance sheet by way of summary,
Six NADPH are formed, three CO_2 set free,
Three ribulose-5-phosphates formed from three of G6P.

One isomerization from the ketose to aldose
Turns ribulose-5-phosphate to the phosphate of ribose,
The other two epimerised, inverted at C3,
Two xylulose-5-phosphates formed (hence called XU5P).

Two carbons from XU5P transferred to the aldose
(Transketolase needs TPP as everybody knows),
Thus three plus seven made to meet transaldolase attack,
Three C's from sedoheptulose the GAP gets back.

Glyceraldehyde-3-phosphate thus becoming F6P
Leaves erythrose-4-phosphate looking for some company,
But XU5P number two has two top C's to spare,
Transketolase negotiates their transfer as a pair.

. . . / . . .

So we've made another F6P, a triose phosphate too,
To see what we have now achieved let's multiply by two,
Four F6P's, two GAP's, by glycolytic tricks,
Give five glucose-6-phosphates, when we started out with six!

December 1978

We must add an addendum, for there's recent work* that shows
A variant in liver cells involving octulose.
If you've just learned the "classic" path, you may think it's a shame,
If it's any consolation though, the end result's the same!

---

*New reaction sequences for the non-oxidative pentose phosphate pathway (J.F.
Williams, P.F. Blackmore and M.G. Clarke), *Biochem. J.* (1978) **176**, 257-282.

MACNAMARA'S BAND

SHAMUS O'CONNOR

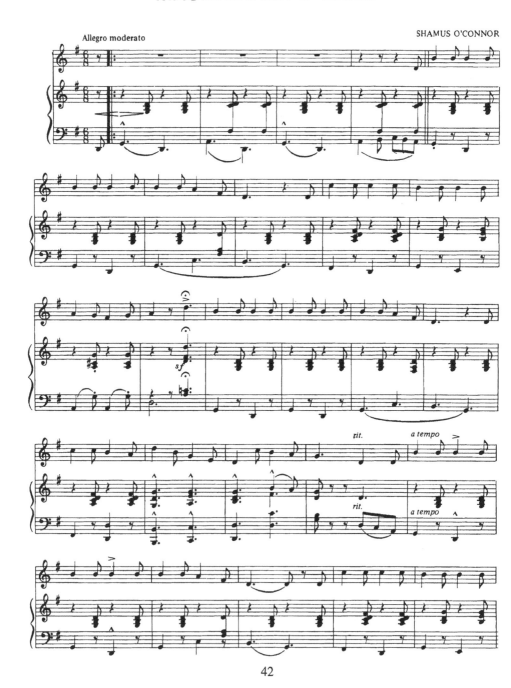

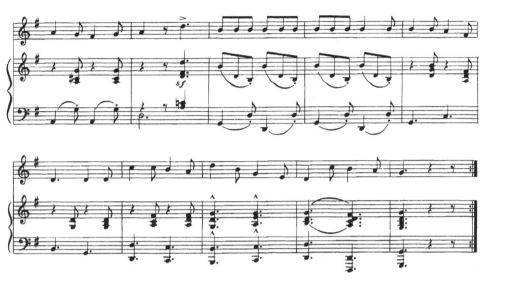

The Pentose Phosphate Pathway

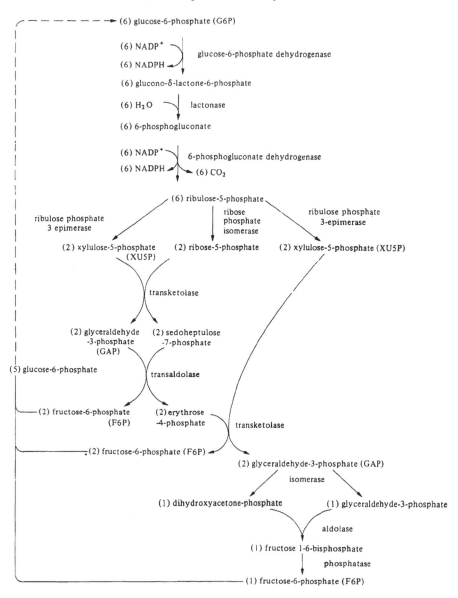

Notes: – (i) Abbreviations have been added when they are used in the song.
(ii) The TPP referred to in the song is thiamine pyrophosphate, the co-factor for transketolase.
(iii) The enzymes of the gluconeogenic steps from GAP have not been given their full names.
(iv) The song, for simplicity (?), starts with 3 X G6P, yielding 2F6P plus 1GAP (+3CO$_2$). Only then is everything doubled to allow for the gluconeogenic steps 2GAP-- $\rightarrow$ F6P.

FATTY ACID BIOSYNTHESIS
(Tune: "Men of Harlech")

If you gobble tagliatelli,
Chicken soup with vermicelli,
You'll acquire a sagging belly—
What's the use of that?
If your intake's calorific,
Guzzling beer till soporific,
Possibly you'll feel terrific,
But you'll end up fat.
Fat against starvation; fat for insulation;
If you sit hard you'll bounce on lard
Which substitutes in females for inflation.
Fat provides when you are needing
Glucogenic when you're seeding
Product of excessive feeding—
Hail adipocyte!

That cell does not believe in spurning
Excess food that it's not burning,
Therefore carbohydrate turning
To an acetyl,
Trapped inside the matrix spaces
CoA esters in such places
Need to show some fancy paces
And a dash of style.
Hence, citrate formation, anion translocation
(The other way, goes malate, say)
And cleavage then reverses condensation,
Acetyl CoA formation
Outside ready for ligation
Now forms by carboxylation
Malonyl CoA.

. . . / . . .

Fatty acid synthetase is
So complex that it amazes
By the subtle interphases
Between every piece.
Twice we find a thiol centre
Through which all new carbons enter
Structured so as to prevent a
Premature release.
First one on the scene I'll say is pantothenyl
On ACP, as we shall see,
A carrier of acyl groups, but meanwhile
There's an outer thiol station
Much involved in condensation,
Starts off with an acylation
By an acetyl.

Firstly, now all that's been stated,
ACPs malonylated,
Which of course is integrated
With CoA release.
Now there is a new ligation
Paid by de-carboxylation,
Acetyl from outer station
Makes a C4 piece.
Really it's quite neat, oh! Nature doesn't veto
What we've just seen, on methylene
Gives ACP with acyl β keto,
ACP now acts as hinging,
Keto acyl is now swinging
Till its keto group it's bringing
To the reductase.

If, when we're metabolizing
It's for biosynthesizing
NADPH arising
Has a ready use.
Pentose phosphate H-extraction,
Also malic enzyme action,
All in cytosolic fraction,
All set to reduce
Keto group reduction, hydroxy construction
On ACP, so never free,
Hydroxy β butyryl production,

Next we swing to dehydration,
Enoyl ACP formation,
Then a new hydrogenation
Saturates the chain.

Acyl fate is now transferal
To free thiols peripheral,
Pantothenyls thus prepare all
For the next attack,
As in circuit we've just ended
Malonyl is apprehended,
ACP again appended,
C4 now passed back,
Bicarb. generating, C6 thus creating,
Again we've got, on β spot,
A keto in the chain we're saturating,
That's reduced, then dehydrated,
Double-bond eliminated,
Now repeat, till we've created
Palmitoyl CoA!

MEN OF HARLECH

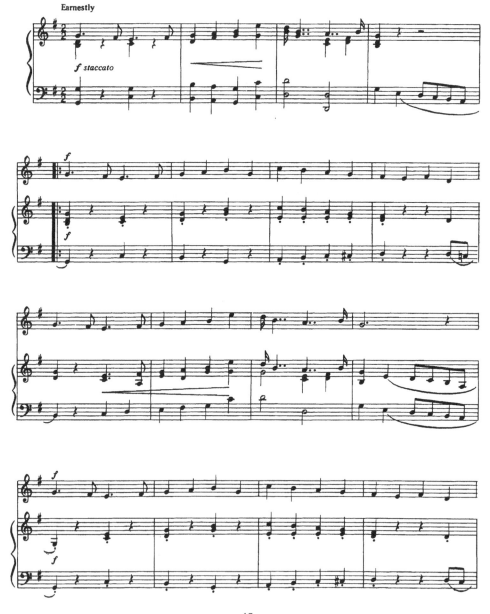

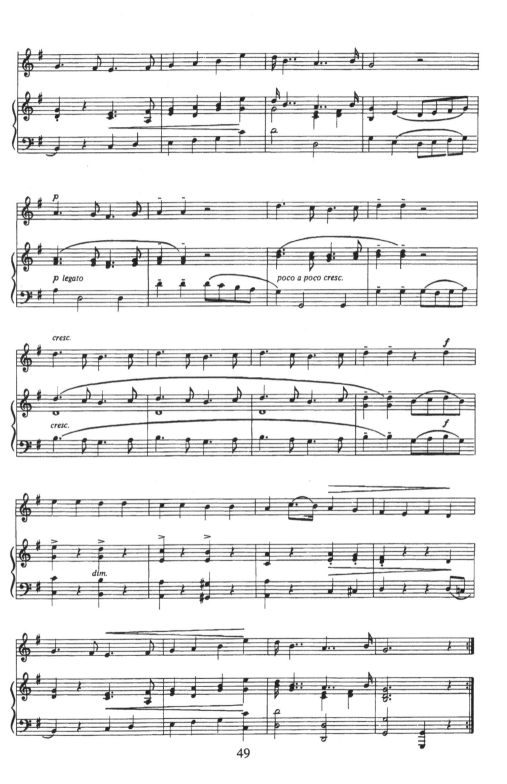

49

Fatty Acid Biosynthesis

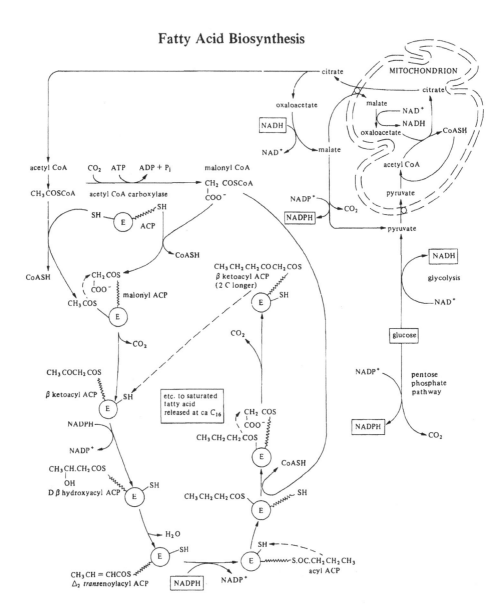

WE'RE HERE BECAUSE UREA
(Tune: "The Bold Gendarmes")

The endogenous repletion of water in the sea
Lets nitrogenous excretion proceed quite easily
For ammonia though toxic is quickly washed away
So fish excrete *(4 times)* the ammonotelic way *(repeat)*.

But new terrestrial creatures to survive where it was dry
Developed metabolic features in order to detoxify,
Since urea is quite soluble and it doesn't make you sick
We each excrete *(4 times)* as a ureotelic *(repeat)*.

When protein breakdown is induced (to make new glucose, say)
Amino acids thus produced give nitrogen away,
Keto acids are acceptors; and oxaloacetate
Transaminates . . . giving rise to aspartate.

Glutamate too may be produced from oxoglutarate
And now that it's been introduced deamination is its fate
For inside each mitochondrion of every liver cell
Is GDH . . . (reducing NAD as well).

Ammonia that's thus set free combined with CO_2
Utilising ATP (and an extra squiggle too)
The effector of the synthetase is acetyl glutamate,
The product formed . . . carbamoylphosphate.

Two amino acid oddities now enter on the scene,
The essential commodities, ornithine and citrulline;
Ornithine starts in the cytosol, citrulline in mitos. free
Then they exchange . . . electrogenically.

Carbamoylphosphate carbamylates the ornithine
So we get a kind of steady state generating citrulline;
Citrulline now is exported, then combined with aspartate
And generates . . . argininosuccinate.

. . . / . . .

That Schiff base condensation utilises ATP
But there is now elimination and fumarate's set free;
Fumarate through citric cycle yields oxaloacetate
That then in turn . . . gives another aspartate.

That cleavage mentioned just before also yielded arginine
And what this pathway's called a cycle for can now readily be seen
For arginine is hydrolysed regenerating ornithine
Which can exchange . . . for another citrulline.

That arginase reaction then also yielded urea
(Aspartate gave one nitrogen, one from ammonia)
And we thus complete the cycle that let us leave the sea,
Sing urea . . . which set the people free.

THE BOLD GENDARMES

arr. G. Todd

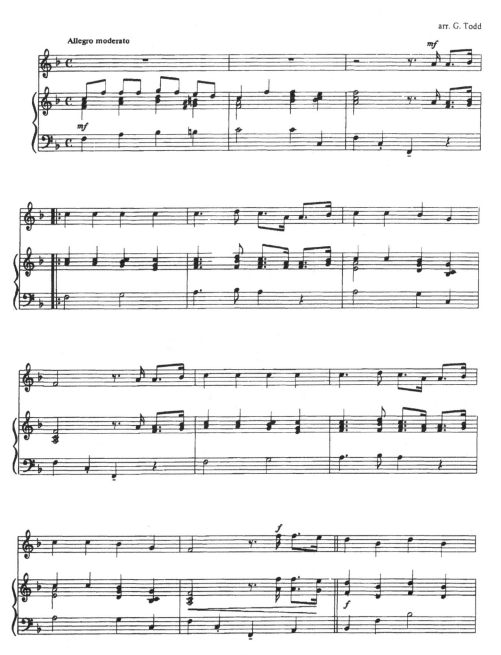

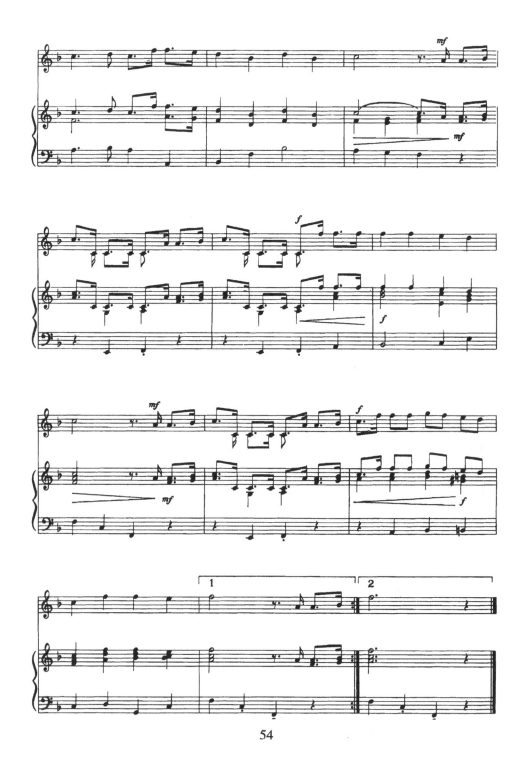

The Urea Cycle

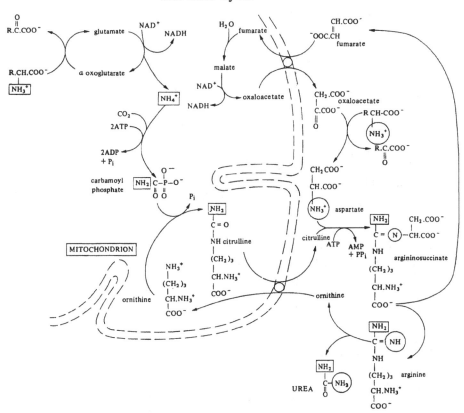

MITOCHONDRION

UREA

55

PROTEIN BIOSYNTHESIS
(Tune: "My Bonny Lies Over the Ocean")

The primary sequence of proteins
Is coded within DNA
On sense strand of the double helix
Coiled antiparallel way.
(Introns and exons, changes post-transcriptional, and all
Glycosylations, don't alter such basics at all).

DNAs read 3 prime to 5 prime
Triplet permutations of base
Degenerate, non-overlapping
Variations occur at third place
(A-T and G-C, the four deoxyribotides, besides
U-A and C-G, complement as nucleotides).

Now DNA acts as a template
For RNA polymerase
Transcribing the genetic message
But in antiparallel phase
(5 prime to 3 prime, that's the new message's way, OK?
Encoded this time in new messenger RNA).

tRNA we now consider
With clover leaf multiple bend
Anticodon length at the bottom
Ad'nine at the free 3 prime end
(From 3 to 5 now, so runs that coding base batch, or patch
Third bases somehow, can wobble a bit when they match).

tRNA now gets as loading
Amino acyl moiety
By way of an enzyme-bound donor
Amino acyl AMP
(Enzyme selective, for each amino acyl load—its mode
Takes the respective tRNA with the right code).

. . . / . . .

The ribosome has two subunits
Differing somewhat in weight,
To start protein synthetic sequence
They firstly must dissociate
(Eukaryotic, to 60S and 40S—unless
Prokaryotic, which are similar but weigh less).

Methionine has as adaptor
That is, as its tRNA,
A species with an anticodon
To code saying 'please start this way'
(Met tRNA binds mRNA AUG, you see,
Factors can now play their roles aided by GTP).

They're complexed all with small subunit
Then larger subunit locks in
Met tRNA on the P site
And translation now can begin
(Next tRNA, with its amino acyl on, stuck on
Binds at the site A, at the very next codon along).

Methionine now is transferred from
Ester binding on tRNA
To form peptide bond with amino
Acyl group tagged on at site A
(Messenger moves on, peptidyl adaptor to P, you see
Still on its codon, Met tRNA falls off free).

New loaded adaptor attaches
At A site, next bit of the code
Peptidyl now is transferred to
Amino of incoming load
(Messenger in train, loads site P with tripeptidyl, in style
Frees site A again, to take next amino acyl).

Thus chain grows from end free amino
Specified by mRNA
'Till there's a termination message
Like UAG or UAA
(Peptides when complete, released to their subsequent fate, they state
And when not replete, ribosomes will dissociate).

. . . / . . .

Translation requires many factors,
Breaks down GTP on the way,
Prokaryotics all start with
N-formyl Met tRNA
(On mRNA, translating in sequential train, again
Polysome array, makes replicates of the same chain).

Student feedback:

Oh golly that was a long saga,
Oh gosh how the scansion was strained,
I've just sung this song to my bonny,
No wonder my bonny looks pained.
Bring back, oh bring back, oh bring back my text book to me, to me,
Bring back, oh bring back plain simple biochemistry.

MY BONNIE

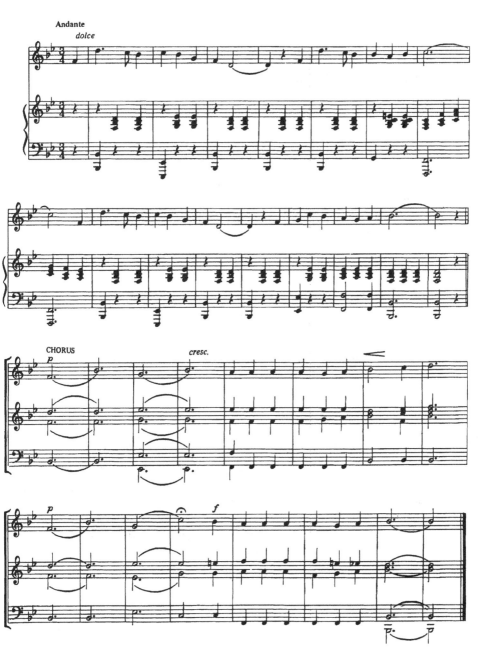

Protein Biosynthesis

A. Transmission of genetic information.

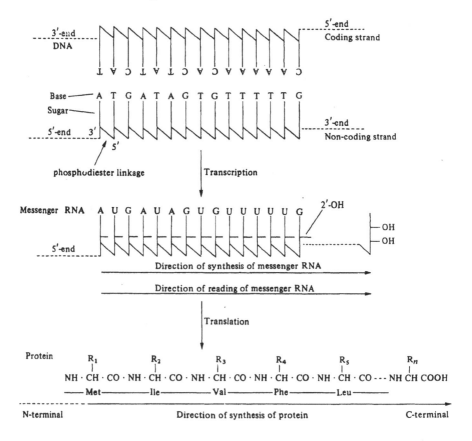

Reproduced with permission from *A Companion to Biochemistry*, Ed. A.T. Bull *et al*, Longman

B. General clover-leaf structure for tRNA.

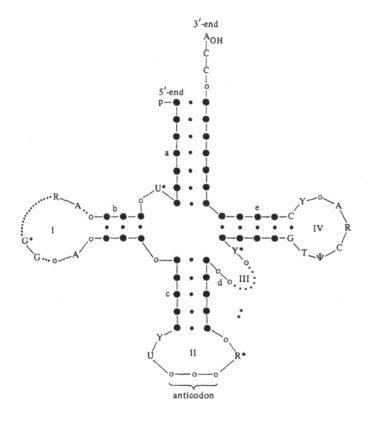

Full circles are H-bonded bases in base pairs. Open circles are bases not in clover-leaf base pairs. H-bonds in base pairs are represented by big dots. R = purine base. Y = pyrimidine base. * indicates that the nucleotide may be modified. Base-paired regions (stems) are numbered a to e and non base-paired bases are in loops I to IV. The dotted part of loops I and III indicate variation on number of nucleotides.

C. Charging of tRNA with an amino acid in a two-step enzymic process.

$$R \cdot \underset{\underset{(+)}{NH_3}}{\overset{\overset{O}{\|}}{CH} \cdot C} - O^{(-)} + ATP \underset{\underset{(Step\ I)}{(A.E.)}}{\overset{Activating\ enzyme}{\longrightarrow}} \left[R \cdot \underset{\underset{(+)}{NH_3}}{\overset{\overset{O}{\|}}{CH} \cdot C} - O - \overset{O^{(-)}}{\underset{O}{\overset{\|}{P}}} - O - CH_2 \cdots \right] + PP_i$$

Aminoacyl-adenylate: activating enzyme complex

A.E.: Aminoacyl-adenylate + tRNA $\xrightarrow[\text{(Step II)}]{}$ $\left[\begin{matrix} tRNA \\ chain \end{matrix} \right]$ $-\overset{O^{(-)}}{\underset{O}{\overset{\|}{P}}} - O - CH_2 \cdots$ + AMP

Overall reaction: Amino acid + ATP + tRNA $\xrightarrow{\text{A.E.}}$ aminoacyl-tRNA + AMP + PP$_i$

D. Scheme for steps so far detected in polypeptide chain initiation.

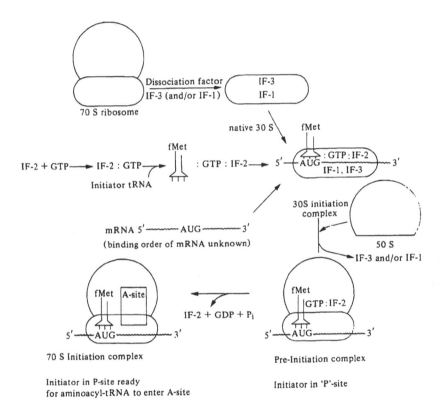

NB. In the case of eukaryotic cells, the ribosome is 80 S, the small subunit 40 S, and the initiating methionyl group is not N-formylated.

E.   Cyclic scheme for peptide bond formation.

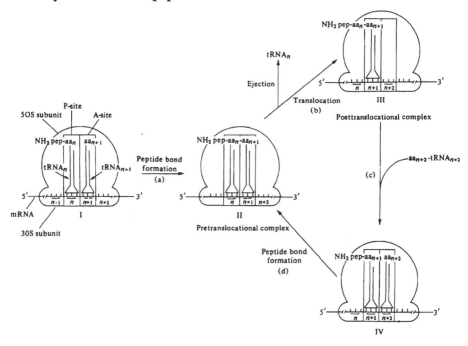

HAEM BIOSYNTHESIS

(Tune: "A Policeman's Lot is not a Happy One")

If you need more haemoglobin for tomorrow – for tomorrow
And your cytochromic store's run out of steam – out of steam
There's a metabolic pathway you should follow – you should follow
Biosynthetic route that leads to haem – leads to haem
In mitochondrion the path commences – path commences
The δ-amino laevulinate way – 'inate way
Glycine decarboxylates when it condenses – it condenses
On the synthetase with succinyl CoA.

Chorus: The most elegant of pathways you could dream – you could dream
For assembling porphyrins and making haem.

Haem inhibiting of that committing start meant – 'itting start meant
Making δ-ALA to meet your needs – meet your needs
Leaving now the mitochondrial compartment – 'al compartment
Condense in pairs as dehydrase succeeds – 'ase succeeds
Porphobilinogen the pyrrole product – pyrrole product
Now condenses head to tail, four to a string – to a string
Three ammoniums are lost forming that adduct – 'ing that adduct
Methylene bridge is thus formed between each ring.

Chorus

Next, linear tetrapyrrole bound to synthase – bound to synthase
In cyclising loses fourth ammonia – 'mmonia
And the synthase and cosynthase acting in phase – acting in phase
Make asymmetric cyclic polymer – polymer
Uroporphyrinogen III created – III created
Side chains don't quite alternate as you'd deduced – you'd deduced
Next all acetates are decarboxylated – 'oxylated
Coproporphyrinogen III is produced.

Chorus

. . . / . . .

Into mitochondrion having migrated – 'ing migrated
Two vinyls first are formed from propionates – propionates
For protoporphyrin IX to be created – be created
Coproporphyrinogen desaturates – 'saturates
Ferrous iron is finally inserted – 'ly inserted
The enzyme now of course ferrochelatase – 'chelatase
So two simple starting substances converted – 'ces converted
To a complex haem which can't fail to amaze!

The most elegant of pathways you could dream – you could dream
For assembling porphyrins and making haem – making haem.

A POLICEMAN'S LOT IS NOT A HAPPY ONE

Sir Arthur Sullivan (from Gilbert and Sullivan's 'Pirates of Penzance')

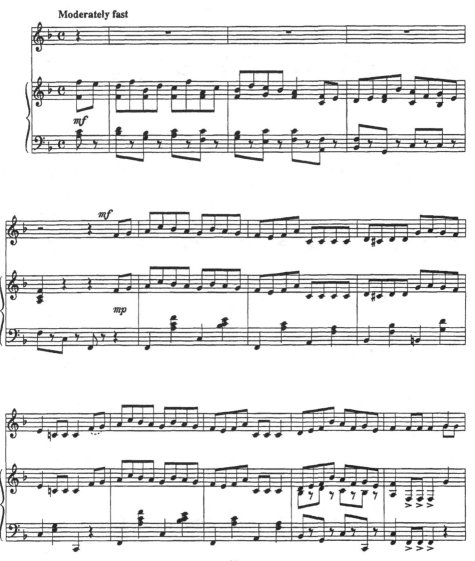

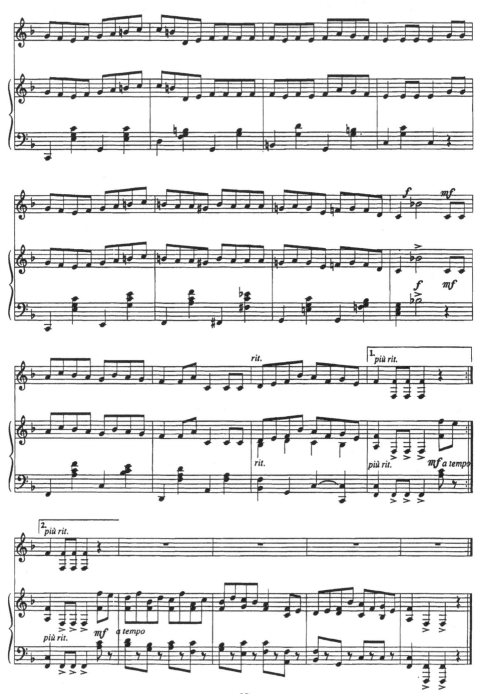

68

Biosynthesis of Haem

METABOLISM OF ODD-NUMBER CARBON FATTY ACIDS

(Tune: "Tit-Willow")

When a cow in its rumen's fermenting the cud
To get sugar, sweet sugar, sweet sugar
It's surprising what products first enter the blood
It's not sugar at all, no not sugar
But it's short fatty acids instead of glucose
That the ruminal bugs have made from cellulose
So the cow has a problem of how to turn those
Into sugar, blood sugar, milk sugar.

Of those short fatty acids the browsing cow gains
Wanting sugar, sweet sugar, sweet sugar
Some have odd carbon numbers in their fatty chains
Unlike sugar, six carbon blood sugar
β oxidation must then come into play
After activation in an ATP way
To become or to yield propionyl CoA
Not yet sugar, blood sugar, milk sugar.

Propionyl CoA then adds on CO_2
Four carbons so far, unlike sugar
The carboxylase using an ATP too
It costs quite a lot to make sugar
Methylmalonyl CoA thus having been made
An isomerase comes along, places to trade
(No ATP needed, bond energy's paid)
We're now on the way towards sugar.

. . . / . . .

That methylmalonyl CoA isomerase
Has B_{12} coenzyme, so sugar
Requires cobalt from pastures on which the cows graze
Those cows that have got to make sugar
From isomerisation, succinyl CoA
Then oxaloacetic, the TCA way
PEP carboxykinase will then come into play
Hooray, the cow now can make sugar.

For once cows have made PEP they are over the worst
To make sugar, sweet sugar, sweet sugar
Glycolytic pathway is simply reversed
NADH needed for sugar
So the cow now has fuel for its timid brain
Can make lactose to sweeten its milking again
Fermented waste product has become the cow's gain
As sugar, sweet sugar, sweet sugar.

TIT-WILLOW

Sir Arthur Sullivan (from Gilbert and Sullivan's 'Mikado')

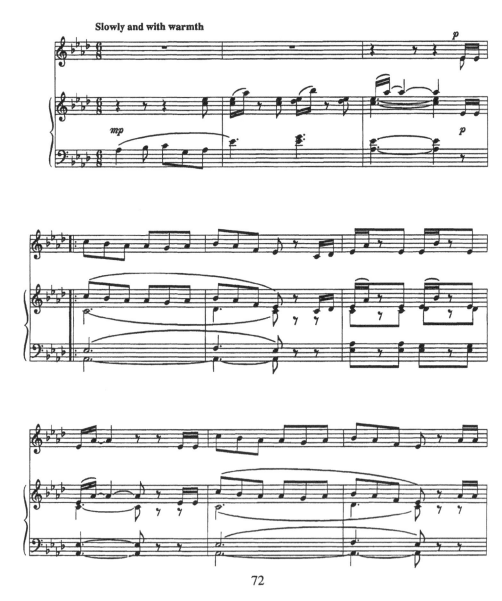

72

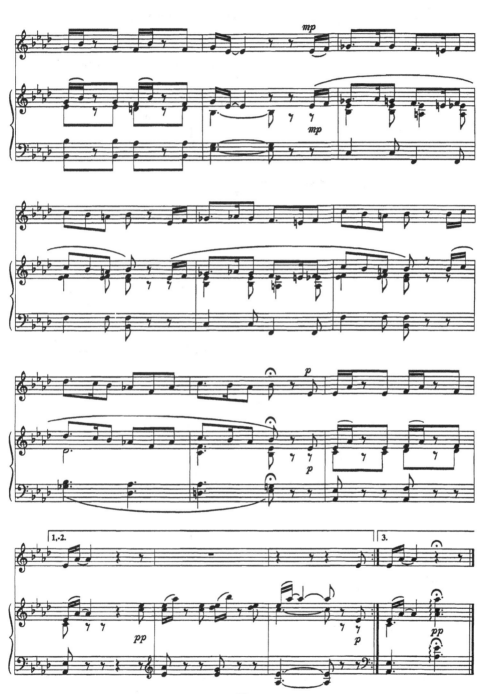

Gluconeogenesis from fatty acids with odd numbers of carbon atoms

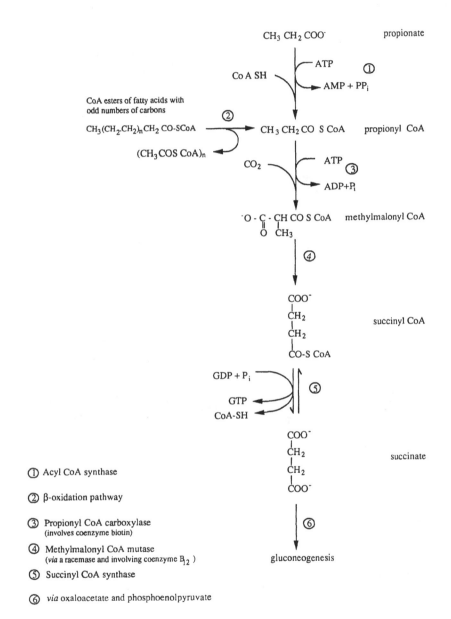

$CH_3 CH_2 COO^-$ propionate

① Acyl CoA synthase

② β-oxidation pathway

③ Propionyl CoA carboxylase
(involves coenzyme biotin)

④ Methylmalonyl CoA mutase
(*via* a racemase and involving coenzyme B_{12})

⑤ Succinyl CoA synthase

⑥ *via* oxaloacetate and phosphoenolpyruvate

REGULATION OF KETOGENESIS
(Tune: "Clementine")

In starvation, diabetes, sugar levels under strain
You need fuel to keep going saving glucose for your brain
Ketone bodies, Ketone bodies, both acetoacetate
And its partner on reduction, 3-hydroxybutyrate.

Glucagon's up, with low glucose, insulin is down in phase
Fatty acids mobilised by hormone-sensitive lipase
Ketone bodies, Ketone bodies, all start thus from white fat cell
Where through lack of glycerol-P, TG making's down as well.

Now transported to the liver, fatty acids activate
Giving CoA thioesters, oxidation is their fate
Ketone bodies, Ketone bodies, because low glycerol-P
Glucagon up, insulin down, stops reversal to TG.

Fatty acyl, CoA level, makes kinase phosphorylate
Acetyl Co-A carboxy-lase to its inactive state
Ketone bodies, Ketone bodies, because glucagon they say
Also blocks carboxylation, lowers malonyl CoA.

Malonyl CoA's a blocker of the key CPT-I
Blocking's off so now the shuttle into mito's is begun
Now we've β oxidation, now we've acetyl CoA
But what's to stop its oxidation via good old TCA?

In starvation, glucose making, stimulating PEP CK
Uses oxaloacetic, also lost another way
Ketone bodies, what is odd is that the oxidation state
Also favours the reduction of OA to give malate.

OA's low now, citrate synthase, thus loses activity
So the flux into the cycle cuts off (temporarily)
Ketone bodies, Ketone bodies, situation thus is this
Acetyl CoA's now pouring into Ketogenesis.

. . . / . . .

It's a tricky little pathway, it's got HMG CoA
In effect it's condensation in a head-to-tailish way
Ketone bodies, Ketone bodies, note the ratio of the pair
Is controlled by NAD to NADH everywhere.

Don't despise them, they're good fuels for your muscles, brain and heart
When your body's overloaded though, that's when your troubles start
Ketone bodies, Ketone bodies, make acetone, lose CO_2
You can breathe those out, but watch out – acidosis does for you!

CLEMENTINE

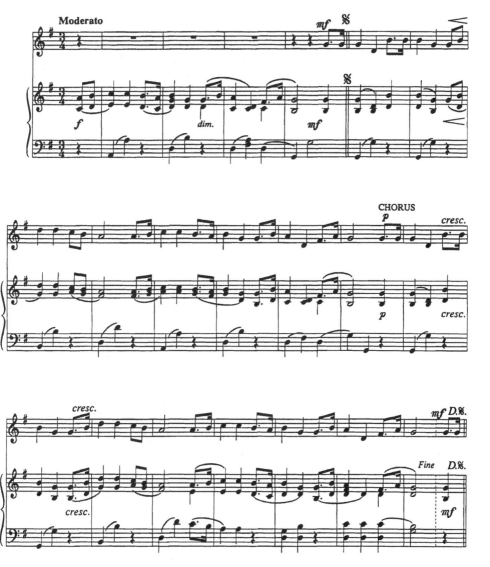

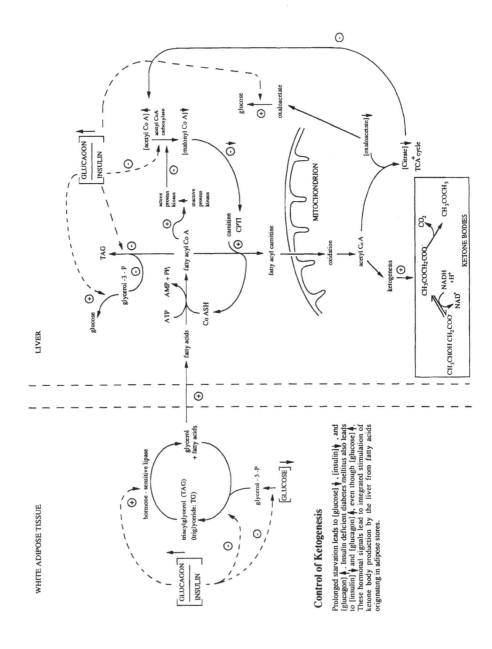

Control of Ketogenesis

Prolonged starvation leads to [glucose]↓, [insulin]↓, and [glucagon]↑. Insulin deficient diabetes mellitus also leads to [insulin]↓ and [glucagon]↑, even though [glucose]↑. These hormonal signals lead to integrated stimulation of ketone body production by the liver from fatty acids originating in adipose stores.

PURINE BIOSYNTHESIS

(Tune: "Camptown Races")

Oh glycine gives C-5 and 4 and N-7
N-1 aspartate what is more, C-6 CO_2
N-3 and 9 from glutamine, amino donor
On tetrahydrofolate's been carbons 8 and 2
Purine origins summarised for you
And starting with ribose-5-phosphate then
We can sing the pathway through.

Add on a pyrophosphate now, at first carbon
Donor is ATP somehow, α-form you see
Committing enzyme on the scene, amido transfer
Amino from glutamine, pyrophosphate free
There's inversion on C-1 moiety
Phosphoribosylamine glycoside
C-Nβ geometry.

Glycine adds on the amino side, splits ATP
Glycinamide nucleotide, next we formylate
Product αN formyl, glycinamide
Donor was N-10 formyl, tet'hydrofolate
(Note that it's still in nucleotidyl state)
Amide's converted to an amidine
With glutamine to donate.

ATP paid as often seen, for that transfer
Makes formyl glycinamidine, ribonucleotide
Dehydration's now its role, and ring closure
5-aminoimidazole, still a nucleotide
And now a CO_2 adds on the C-4 side
Then aspartate adds, makes carboxylate
Succinocarboxamide.

. . . / . . .

79

As in the ornithine cycle then, (to arginine)
Carboxamide keeps nitrogen, loses fumarate
5-aminoamidazole, carboxamide
Takes formyl group that adds on whole, and (no need to state)
N-10 formyltetrahydrofolate
Was donor sending 5-amino group
To formylamino fate.

A dehydration follows now, and ring closure
We've made a purine ring somehow, inosate (IMP)
This pathway's gone on far too long, dooh-dah, dooh-dah
You'll have to write your own sweet song, (done quite easily)
To transform hypo-xanthine moiety
To adenine and guanine counterparts
AMP and GMP.

CAMPTOWN RACES

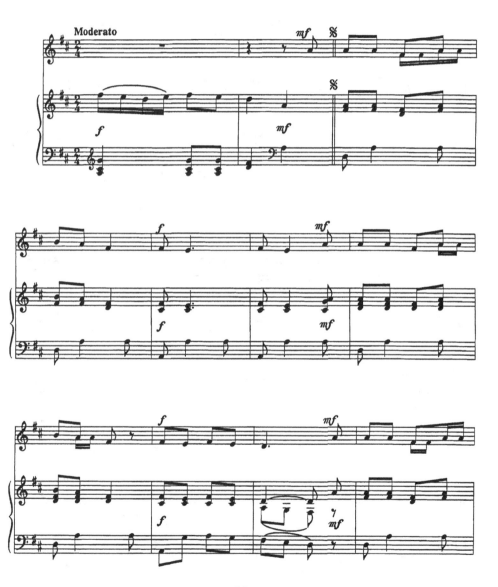

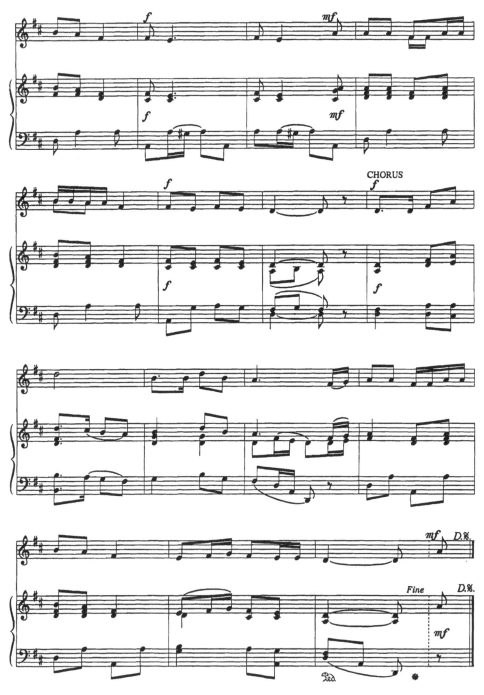

Purine Biosynthesis

PRPP: 5-phosphoribosyl-1-pyrophosphate
PRA: 5-phosphoribosylamine
GAR: glycinamide ribonucleotide
FGAR: formylglycinamide ribonucleotide
FGAMR: formylglycinamidine ribonucleotide
AIR: 5-aminoimidazole ribonucleotide
ACIR: 5-amino-4-carboxy-imidazole ribonucleotide
SAICAR: N-succinylo-5-aminoimidazole-4-carboxamide ribonucleotide
AICAR: 5-aminoimidazole-4-carboxamide ribonucleotide
FAICAR: N-formyl-5-aminoimidazole-4-carboxamide ribonucleotide

(ribose-5-phosphate)

ATP
AMP

(PRPP)

glutamine
glutamate
PP$_i$

(PRA)

glycine
ATP
ADP + P$_i$

(GAR)

ribose - phosphate

N^{10} formyl -
H$_4$ folate
H$_4$ folate

(FGAR)

ribose - phosphate

glutamine
glutamate
ATP
ADP + P$_i$

(FGAMR)

ribose - phosphate

ATP
ATP + P$_i$

(AIR)

ribose - phosphate

CO_2

(ACIR)

ribose - phosphate

aspartate
ATP
ADP + P$_i$

(SAICAR)

ribose - phosphate

fumarate

(AICAR)

ribose - phosphate

N^{10} formyl -
H$_4$ folate
H$_4$ folate

(FAICAR)

ribose - phosphate

H_2O

inosinic acid
(IMP)

ribose - phosphate

AMP   GMP

83

CHOLESTEROL BIOSYNTHESIS

(Tune: "Cwm Rhondda")

Vital for membrane formation
Precursor of hormones too
Bile salts from its oxidation
Cholesterol is good for you
Atheroma? carcinoma?
Despite those hazards that you've read (and heard said)
Without it you'd be surely dead.

Cholesterol, it's been suggested
(Possibly it's really so)
Ensures the more that is ingested
The less assembled *de novo*
Despite its size, it's synthesised
Entirely out of acetyl (that's the style!)
Your liver makes it all the while.

The pathway we can say commences
With three acetyl CoA
One by one each then condenses
In the ketogenic way
Aceto acetyl acts as
Product that is on the way (you could say)
En route to HMG CoA.

Now comes the enzyme that's committing
(Controlled perhaps by feedback loop)
CoA from the end it's splitting
Reducing twice carboxyl group
OH formation oxidation
Of NADPH times two (yes, it's true)
You've mevalonate when you're through.

. . . / . . .

That C-five OH now acceptor
Phosphorylation is its fate
As intermediate you detect a
5-phosphomevalonate
More addition that position
Costing second ATP (not for free)
5-pyrophospho product see!

Transient third phosphorylation
At OH on carbon three
Causes decarboxylation
As the phosphate splits off free
Thus you're making no mistaking
Species to polymerise (happy sighs!)
Reactive and the proper size.

Isopentenyl pyrophosphate
(Branched, five carbon as you'd thought)
Isomerises to its soul mate
The dimethylallyl sort
Head and tail seize without fail these
Two condense to a C-ten (shout 'Amen!')
Geranyl pyrophosphate then.

Geranyl is now transferred to
Isopentenyl third in line
Gives C-fifteen now referred to
As farnesyl, (we're doing fine)
Head to heading P-P shedding
Presqualene ester thus produced (we've deduced)
All ready now to be reduced.

NADPH reductant
Second P-P leaving too
C-thirty squalene resultant
(Three to lose before we're through)
Let us now praise oxygenase
That forms the 2, 3 epoxide (swell with pride!)
With several factors on the side.

. . . / . . .

Methyl shifts are now concerted
Hydrides move along the chain
To lanosterol converted
Suddenly four rings we gain
Ring arounding quite astounding
Catalysed by a cyclase (to amaze)
Within the microsomal phase.

Three methyls eliminated
(C-fourteen and two C-four)
Side chain now is saturated
And in B-ring what is more
Bonds are changing, rearranging
Shift to 5, 6 from 8, 9 (which is fine)
Cholesterol, at last you're mine.

CWM RHONDDA

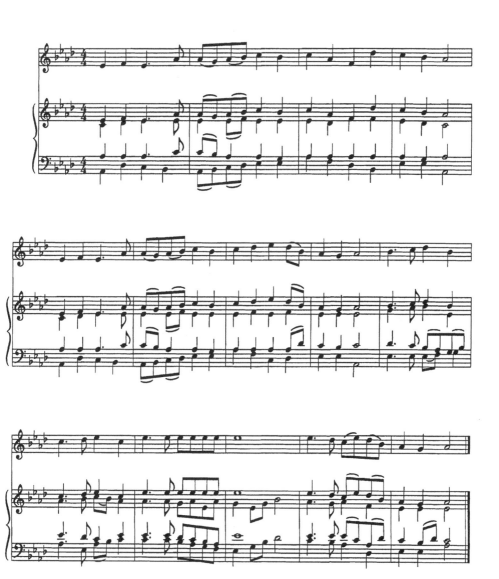

Biosynthesis of Squalene

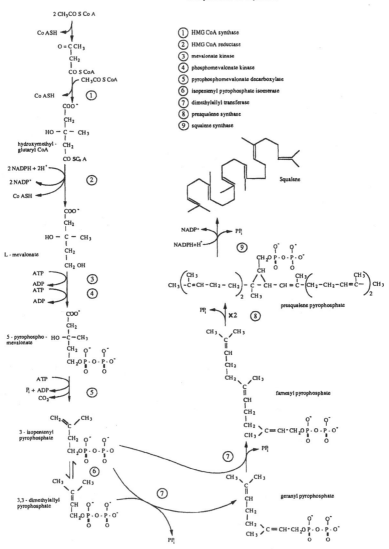

1. HMG CoA synthase
2. HMG CoA reductase
3. mevalonate kinase
4. phosphomevalonate kinase
5. pyrophosphomevalonate decarboxylase
6. isopentenyl pyrophosphate isomerase
7. dimethylallyl transferase
8. presqualene synthase
9. squalene synthase

Conversion of Squalene to Cholesterol

(Outline only; details not covered in song.)

① Squalene monoxygenase (requires molecular oxygen and several co - factors).

② Cyclase (squalene expoxide lanosterol - cyclase)

③ Loss of three methyl groups; saturation of side chain double bond

④ Saturation of 7, 8 double bond

89

A CAUTIONARY CAROL
(Tune: "Good King Wenceslas")

Winter solstice celebrate! Hail the festive season!
Wise men cease to cerebrate! Take a rest from reason!
Super ego is defined (Ellis & Karminski[1])
As that part of human mind soluble in whisky.

But beware for ethanol at levels elevated
In liver cells, in cytosol, is dehydrogenated
NADH to NAD the ratio's distorted
There's aldehyde toxicity (as recently reported[2]).

With NADH levels great, your lactate is frustrated
It can't go to pyruvate to be carboxylated
And sad to say that furthermore, and in that same connection
The poise of acids at C_4 is in malate's direction.

Oxaloacetate is low, carboxykinase slowing
PEP formation *de novo* no longer can keep going
Why this is a menace is manifest quite clearly
Gluconeogenesis grinds to halt (or nearly).

You may blame the awful toll of hangover sensation
To some higher alcohol, or simple dehydration
But don't forget that in one sense, beer, gin or brew illicit
Have metabolic consequence that's common and implicit.

Blood sugar low, the liver fat, they're also calorific
The moral therefore of all that is though we feel terrific
As we imbibe this Christmastide, our life span's getting shorter
But whilst we're waiting till we've died – go easy on the water!

---

1 Actually, I've lost the reference card. Look them up in *Index Medicus* if you're really
  interested.
2 Not by Ellis & Karminski.

GOOD KING WENCESLAS LOOKED OUT

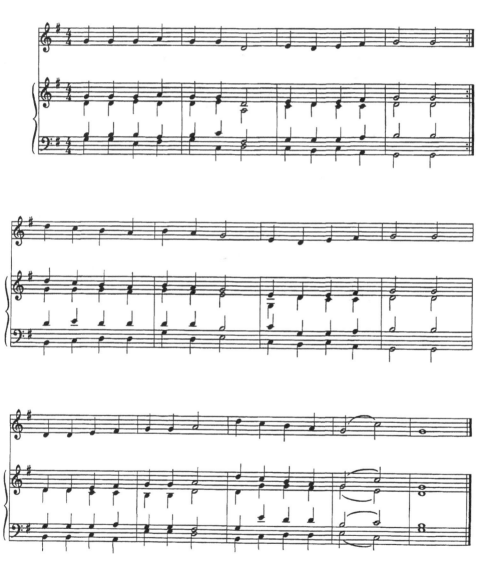

Metabolism of Ethanol

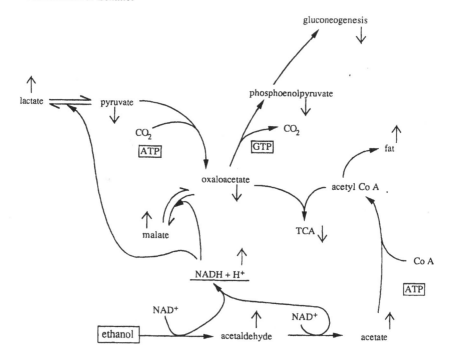

Printed in the United States
by Baker & Taylor Publisher Services